" a glow that comes from growing, not perfecting"

The real glow of Pregnancy

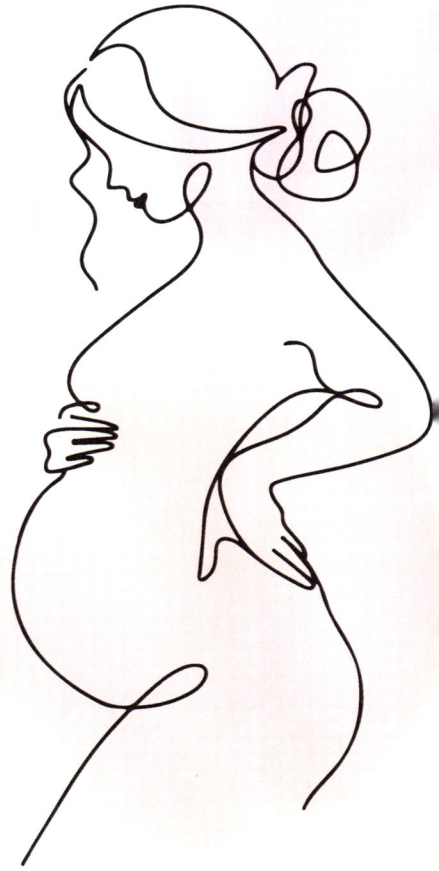

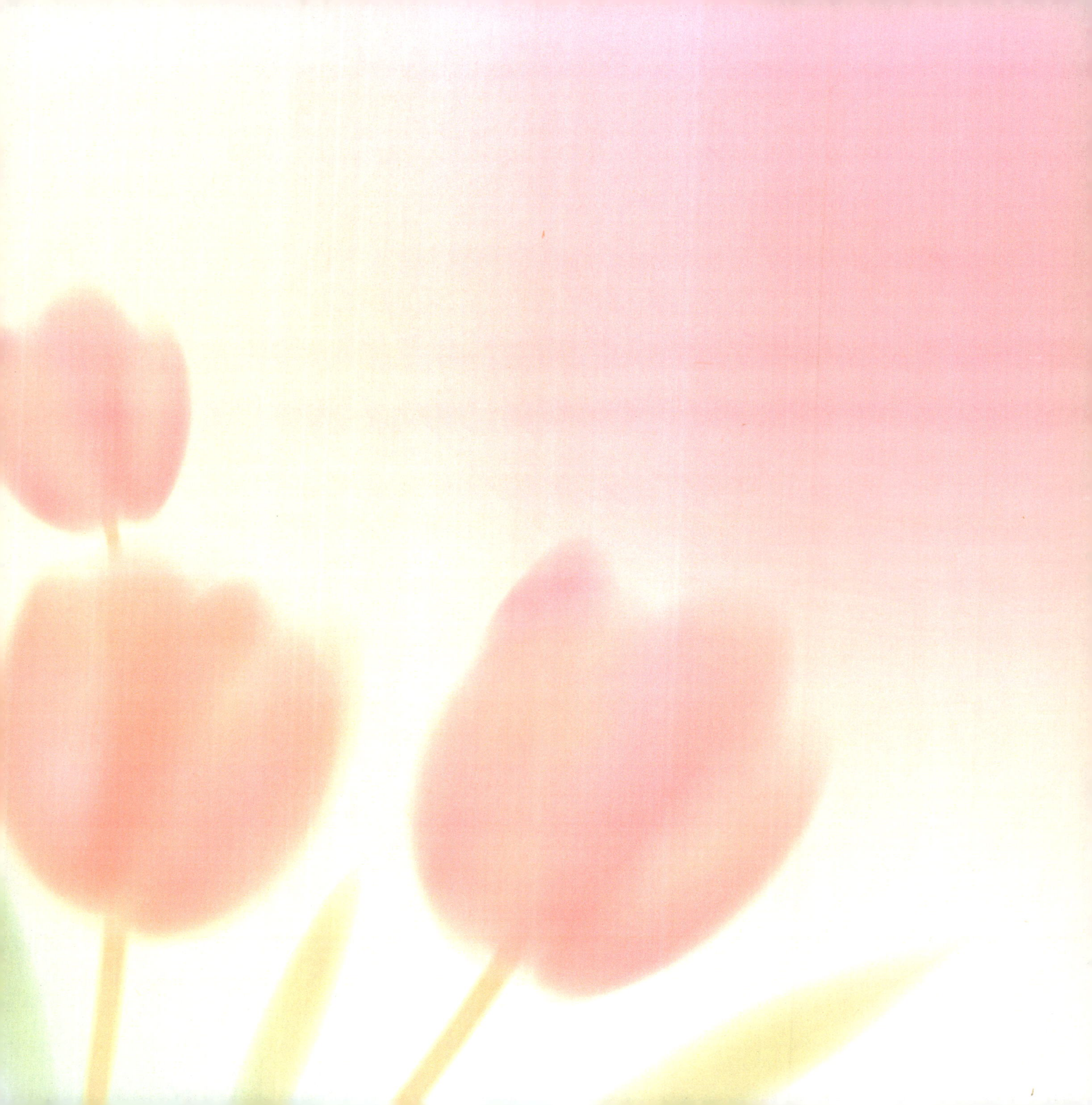

The Real glow of Pregnancy

written by Zandra Mae Cochrane

ISBN: 978-1-7644630-8-9
Printed in Australia
First edition, 2025

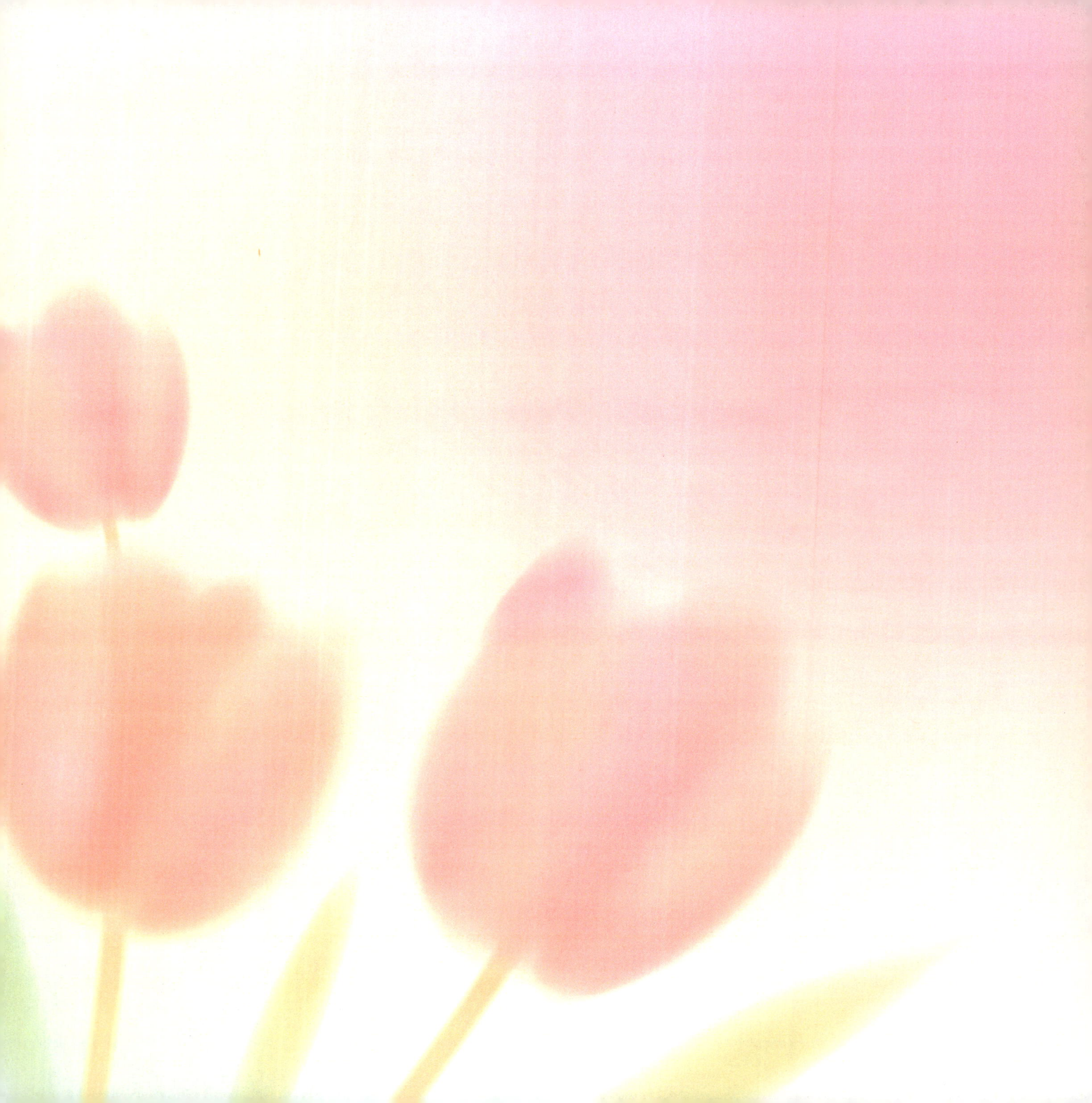

To the mothers who glow through joy, tears, change, and courage.

This is for you...

For every woman who has ever wondered if she was glowing.

You always were...

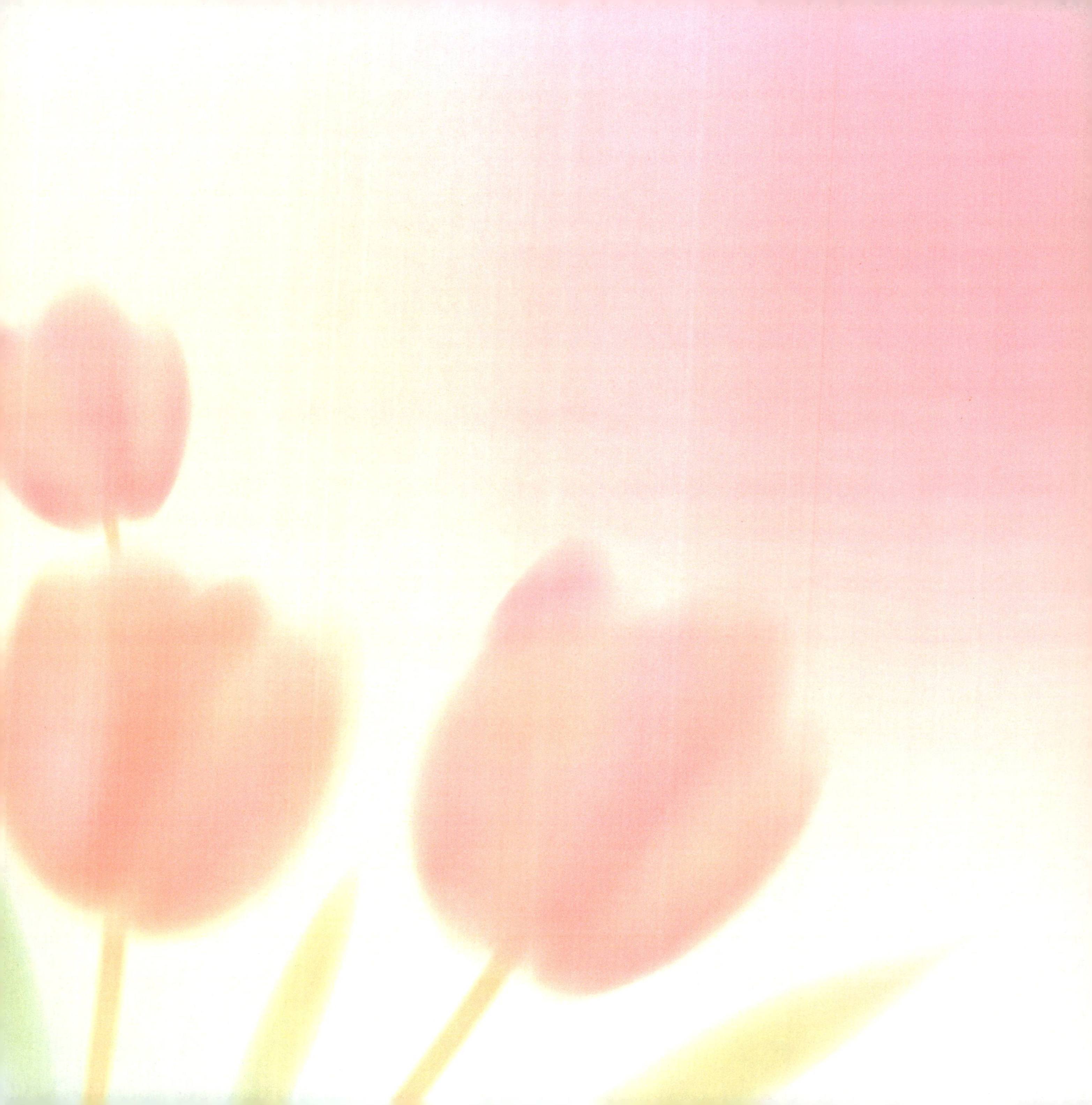

People often say that pregnancy comes
with a glow —
a shine on the skin, a sparkle in the eyes,
a perfect bump,
a beauty that looks effortless and bright.
But not every glow looks the same,
and not every glow shines on the surface

NOR

It isn't always seen in the mirror.

Some women glow with smooth skin and blooming or radiant cheeks...
and some glow through maybe pimples, acne, dry skin, swelling, hormones that paint their faces differently every day and the softness of that change.

Some women stay toned and light on their feet...

and some glow through curves, weight, and the strength of the body carrying life and growth they never expected.

Some women glow in fitted dresses and perfect maternity outfits... and some glow in stretchy pants, loose shirts, and whatever brings comfort and not tight in a day.

Some women glow with endless energy
and excitement...
and some glow go through with slow
mornings or naps, exhaustion, heavy legs,
and the victory of simply getting out of
bed
with quiet breaths.

Some women glow with ease and comfort...
while some glow through nausea,
backaches, pelvic pains, heartburn,
and nights spent trying to find one
comfortable position.

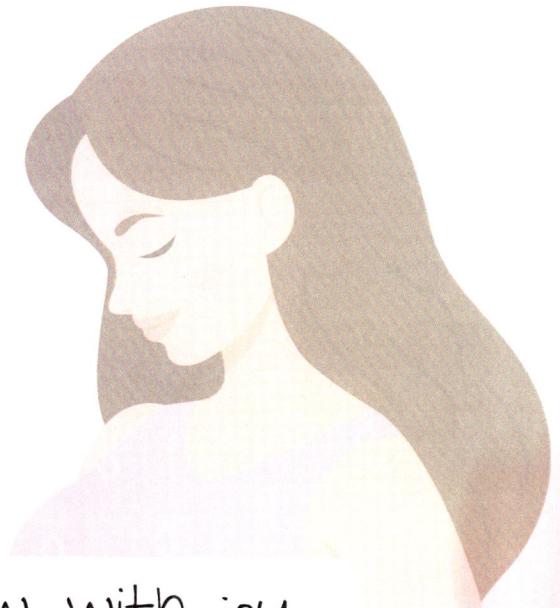

Some women glow with joy...
and some glow through tears, mood
swings, fears, and the courage to feel
everything without an apology and keep
going.

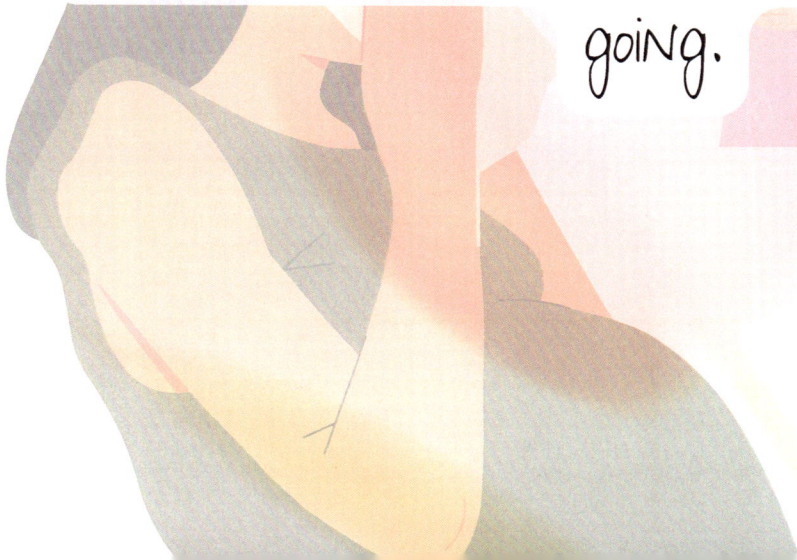

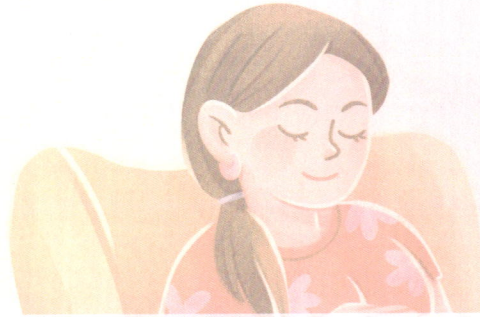

Some women glow with a village around them...
and some glow alone, discovering and finding their own strength they never had.

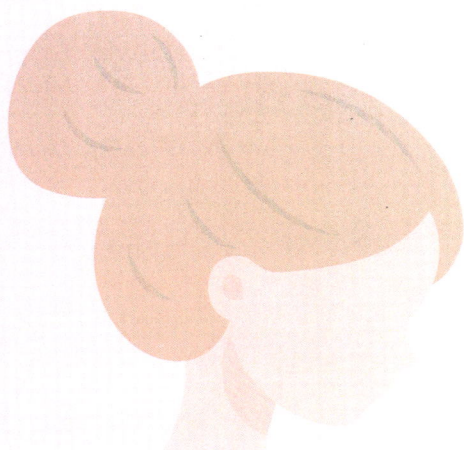

Some women glow with calm...
and some glow through worry,
overthinking,
and the quiet fear of wanting to do
everything right.

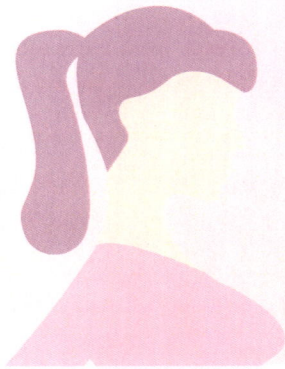

Some women feel instantly connected...
and some glow through slow unfolding
of motherhood, gentle bonding,
and learning to love deeply they
haven't met yet.

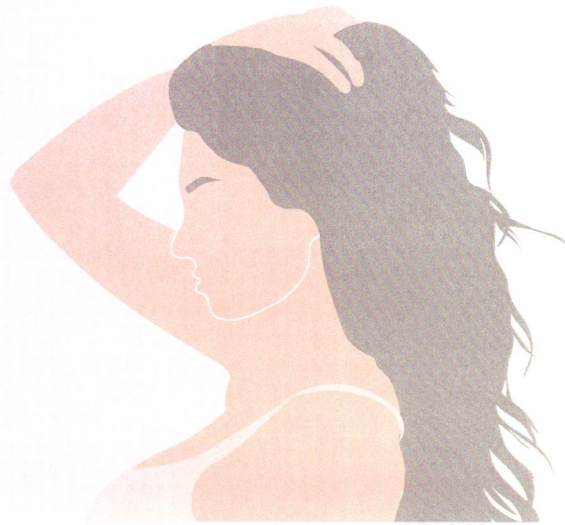

The glow is not in the mirror...
it's in the heart, the body, the
becoming.

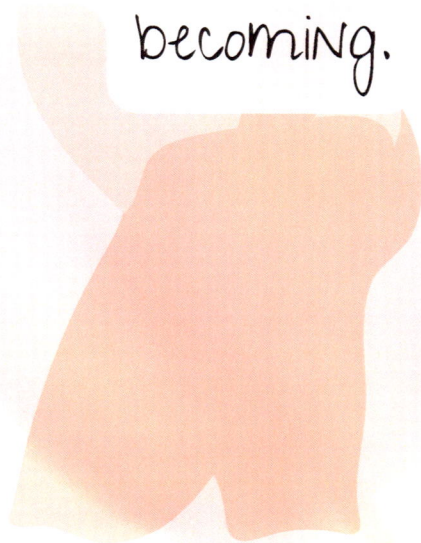

The real glow isn't always visible—
it's in the heartbeat she carries,
the changes she survives,
the love she grows in silence.

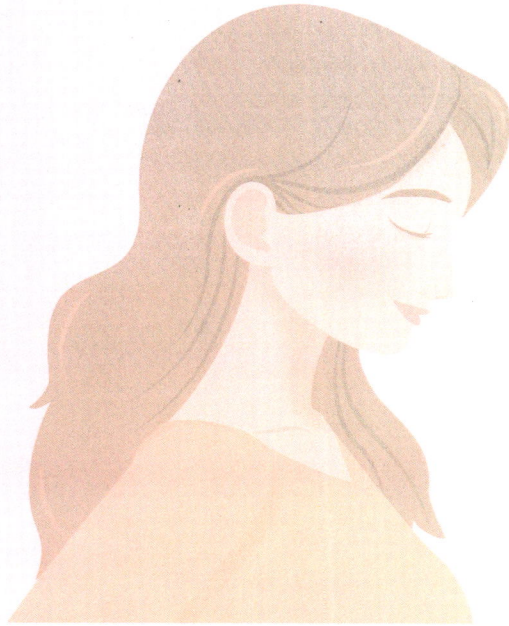

It's in the life growing quietly inside —
a light only she can feel.

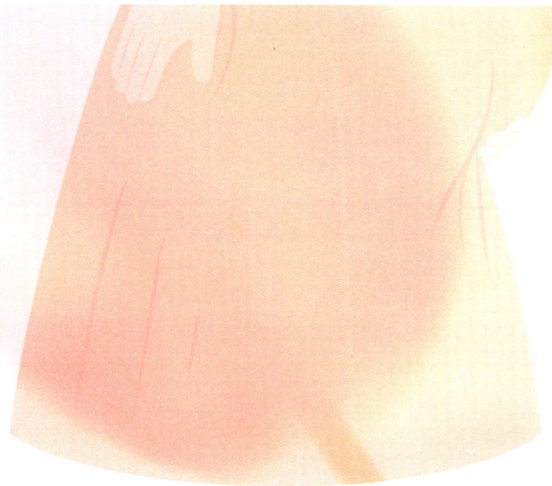

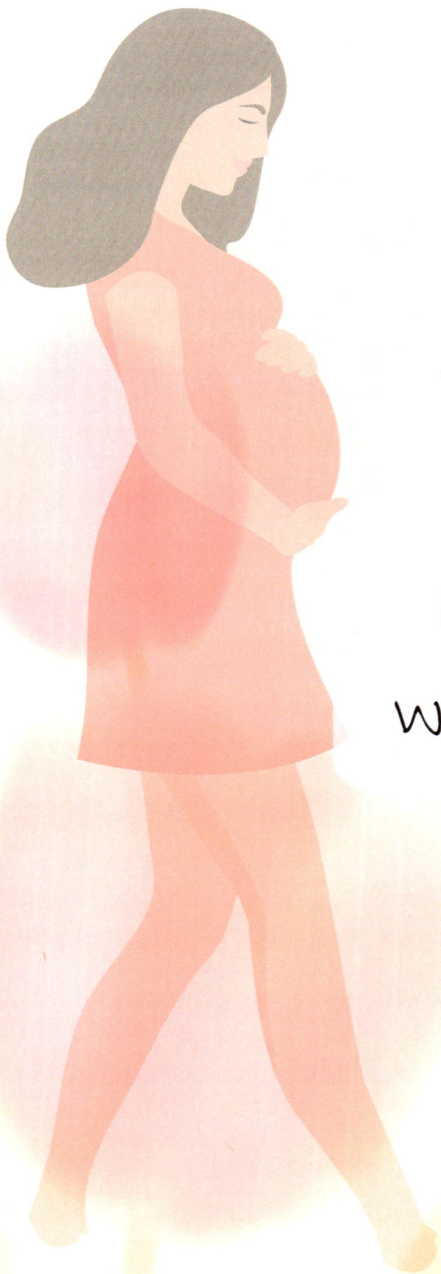

The glow is not perfection.
The glow is transformation
It's becoming someone new
while still holding on to who she
was...

No two pregnancies look the same.

Every glow is unique and real
Every journey is valid.
Every change is real.
Every glow is different—
and
every glow is true.

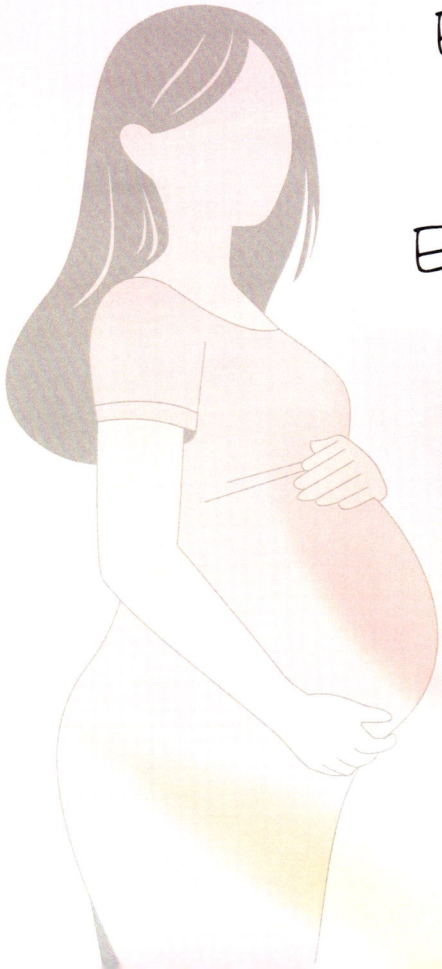

You are glowing—
in your strength,
in your softness,
in your courage,
in your becoming.

Even on the days you don't feel
it.

Your glow doesn't end here.
It grows with you,
into motherhood,
into love,
into every version of who you are
becoming.

Pregnancy is not a single story.
It is a thousand different experiences held inside one body.
Some days feel beautiful.
Some days feel heavy.
Some days feel nothing like the glow people talk about.

But every day, you are growing a life —
and that is a glow no mirror can measure.

This is for every woman who has ever felt unseen,
unprepared, imperfect, or unsure.
Your glow is real.
Your journey is enough.
And you are more radiant than you know.

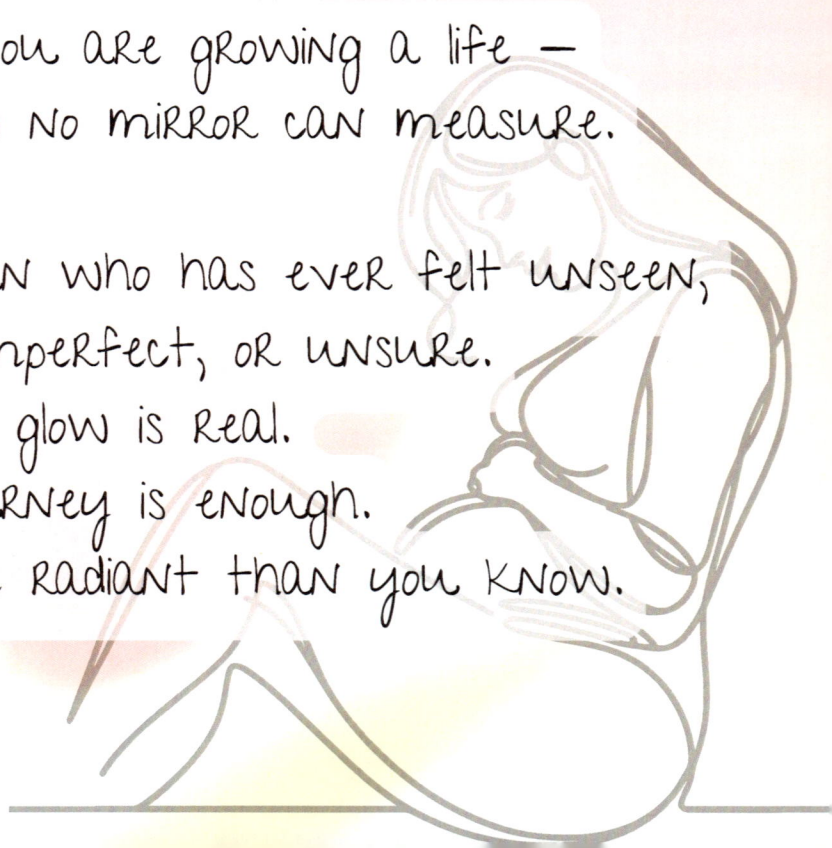

Daily Reminders for you . . .

You are allowed to rest.
You are allowed to slow down.
You are allowed to feel everything.
Your body is working harder than
anyone can see.

Honor it. Listen to it. Trust it.
You don't have to glow on the outside to
be glowing within.
Your glow is in your strength, your
softness, your becoming.

Every change has a purpose.
Every feeling has a place.
Every day, you are doing enough.
You are growing a life —
and that alone is extraordinary.
Be gentle with yourself today.
You deserve it.

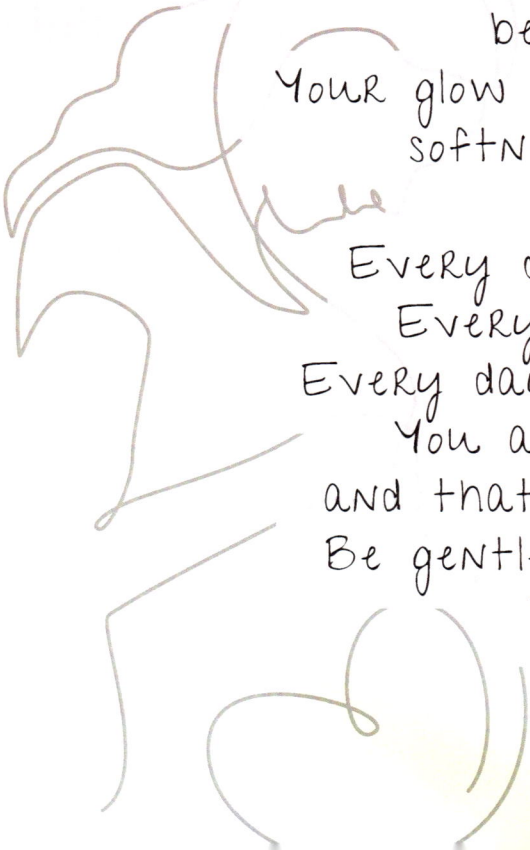

Let's Connect!

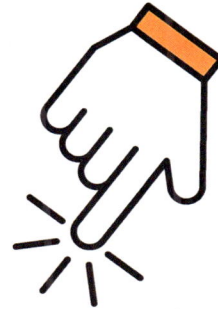

Create with Zandy

COLOURFUL STORIES FOR GROWING HEARTS

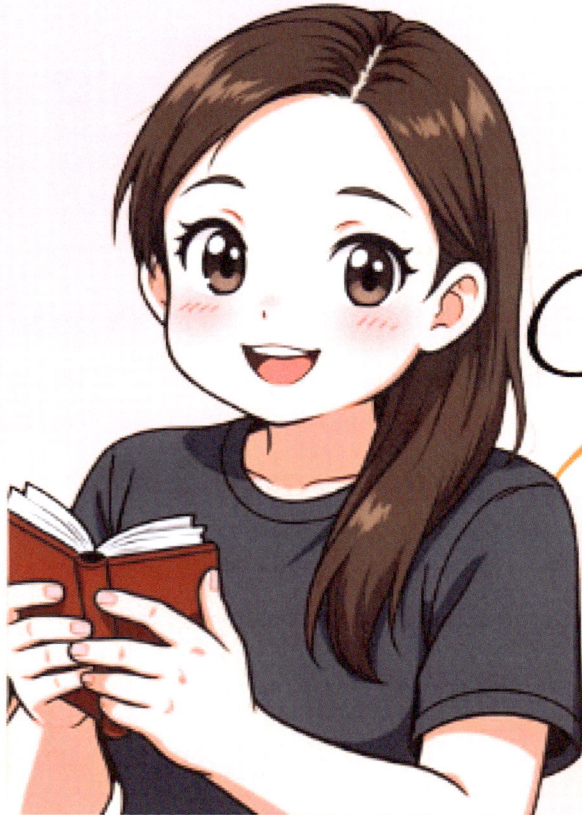

📷 @CREATEWITHZANDY

🌐 ZANDRAMAECOCHRANEBOOKS.COM

✉️ ZANDRAMAECOCHRANE@GMAIL.COM

📞 0432955276

Scan Me

Zandra Mae is a Filipina migrant, educator, and multi-genre author whose work celebrates courage, belonging, and the quiet strength found in everyday life. She writes stories that honor real emotions, real bodies, and real journeys—especially those often overlooked or softened for the world's comfort.

As a mother, and creative writer, Zandra brings a gentle honesty to her writing. Her books blend poetry, reflection, and lived experience, offering comfort and empowerment to readers of all ages.

The Real Glow in Pregnancy was born from her desire to redefine what it means to "glow" during pregnancy—not as perfection, but as transformation.

Through her words, she hopes every woman feels seen, supported, and reminded that her glow is real, even on the days she can't find it in the mirror.

Zandra lives in Perth, Western Australia, where she continues to write stories that uplift families, women, and migrants, turning her own journey of resilience into a source of light for others.

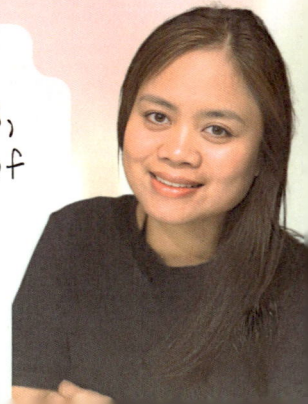

Pregnancy is often described as a time of glowing skin, perfect bumps, and effortless beauty.

But the real glow isn't found in flawless photos or smooth, shining faces. It lives in the quiet courage of change. In the softness that grows with every new curve. In the strength that rises through exhaustion, swelling, tears, and joy. In the love forming long before birth.

The Real Glow in Pregnancy is a gentle, poetic celebration of every woman's journey — the easy ones, the messy ones, the magical ones, and the ones that don't look "glowy" at all.
A reminder that you are radiant not because you are perfect, but because you are becoming.

This book is a warm embrace for every mother-to-be:
a gift of truth, tenderness, and the glow that comes from growing

www.ingramcontent.com/pod-product-compliance
Lightning Source LLC
Chambersburg PA
CBRC091537260326
41914CB00021B/1639